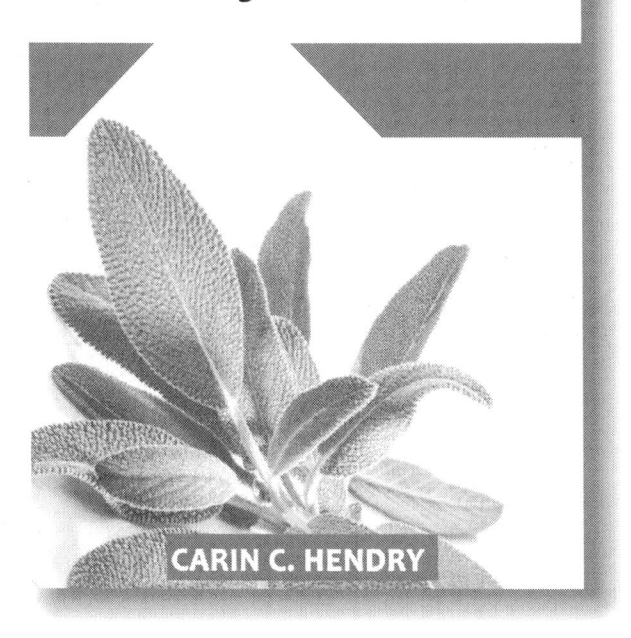

DR. SEBI

How To Naturally Detox The Liver, Reverse Diabetes And High Blood Pressure Through Dr. Sebi Alkaline Diet

CARIN C. HENDRY

DR. SEBI:

How To Naturally Detox The Liver, Reverse Diabetes And High Blood Pressure Through Dr. Sebi Alkaline Diet

Carin C. Hendry

© **Copyright Carin C. Hendry 2019**

All right reserved.

No part of this book may be reproduced, transmitted or stored in a retrieval system in any form or by any means, electronic, mechanical, recording or otherwise without the prior permission of the author.

Dedication

Specially dedicated to all vegans and faithful Sebians.

TABLE OF CONTENT

Dr. Sebi: 2

How To Naturally Detox The Liver, Reverse Diabetes And High Blood Pressure Through Dr. Sebi Alkaline Diet 2

© Copyright Carin C. Hendry 2019 3

Dedication 4

Introduction 8

Chapter [1] 13

How To Naturally Reverse Your Diabetes: The Eat To Live Plan Of Dr. Sebi Natural Food Guide To End Diabetes 13

Chapter [2] 23

Best Natural Foods For Liver Health And Alkaline Diets From Dr. Sebi's Nutritional Food Guide List 23

Chapter [3] 31

Exceptional Strategies Of Dr. Sebi's High Blood Pressure Diet, How To Lower Symptoms Of High Blood Pressure, And What Causes Hypertension....................................31

Chapter [4] 45

Dr. Sebi Electric Food List 45

Note From The Auhor 54

Check Out My Other Similar Books: 56

You don't have to
eat less, you just have to
eat right.

Dr. Sebi Rest in Power

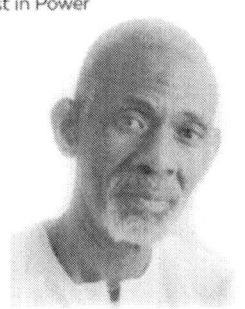

INTRODUCTION

Dr. Sebi was a Honduran man with a very humble beginning and was known and addressed as an herbalist, pathologist or a naturalist in different regions of the world; he left the biosphere in 2016. Indeed, it is true that he is no longer in our midst today, but his self-invented and established effective traditional therapy for diabetes, hypertension and organ cleansing is still helping millions of people with these conditions around the world. He created great strides in the world of natural health and wellness with the creation of his specialized diet.

Dr. Sebi said that there were six fundamental food groups: live, raw, dead, hybrid, genetically modified, and drugs, but his diet basically cut out all the food groups except live and raw food, thereby encouraging dieters to eat as closely to a raw vegan diet as possible.

These foods include foods like naturally grown fruits and vegetables, along with whole grains.

He has the believed that raw and live foods were "electric," which fought the acidic food waste in the body. So, with his approach to eating, Dr. Sebi established a list of foods that he deliberated to be the best for his diet.

Sticking to Dr Sebi's Diet and Food List to cure these diseases can be challenging if you eat out a lot. Consequently, you need to get used to making lots of meals at home.

To help with this, this book was born so as to give you all of the information you need to eat right and the type of herbs to eat to live healthy.

This way you do not have to put too much thought into what you have to eat and the less thought you have to put into the diet, the easier it will become to stick to it.

This great herbalist during his lifetime cured a lot of diseased people and even after his death, he left an exceptional knowledge of holistic healing for diabetes, hypertension and organ cleansing. You too can be inspired from his life and the approach he perceived various terminal diseases. However, you might be worried about treating the above mentioned diseases, right?

Of course, diabetes, hypertension are annoying health conditions that have no remedy in allopathy. This is the reason people are trying several different alternative medicines. Those who are new to this approach of eating are trying them to get total cure, while others already practicing this are just hoping to avoid the side effects of antiviral drugs. Diabetes, hypertension and toxins have without doubt created many health problems in the lives of millions of people, but now is the time you should think about curing it rather than treating.

Chapter [1]

HOW TO NATURALLY REVERSE YOUR DIABETES: THE EAT TO LIVE PLAN OF DR. SEBI NATURAL FOOD GUIDE TO END DIABETES

Diabetes mellitus is undoubtedly one of the fastest killing illnesses in America. This illnesses is caused when the kidney or the pituitary hormone cannot function effectively. The widespread of this disease has been attributed to a slight change otherwise referred to as a defect in the pancreas insulin production. Glucose and insulin are intertwined and being that the body cannot process glucose on its own, it needs insulin to help break down the ingested glucose. Diabetes has its origin rooted in ancient Greek, with its meaning being "pass through" or "flow through". A meaning which has been attributed to how often diabetes sufferers need to ease themselves.

On the other hand, the word mellitus means sweet. In short, diabetes mellitus (type 1, called insulin dependent diabetes) makes it impossible for the pancreas to produce the insulin needed to process the glucose in the body. Type 2 diabetes (insipidus diabetes, called non-insulin-dependent diabetes) also bring about the same flaw as the type 1 with the difference being that the pancreas produces enough insulin which the body finds it hard to process.

The forest not only hides man's enemies but it's full of man's medicine, healing power and food.
~African Proverb

What can make us develop diabetes mellitus?

- Stress
- Obesity
- Pregnancy

Some types of drugs:

- Adrenal corticosteroids
- Thiazide diuretics
- Phenytoin

High sugar diet:

- Sugar

- White flour
- Candy
- Foods containing processed sugar

Natural cures for diabetes:

The habit of over eating and eating late in the night should be stopped as it induces diabetes and makes the condition worse in people who already have it. Instead of depending on conventional everyday food, a diet of high fiber and high carbohydrates should be considered. This diet gradually eliminates the need for insulin. Protein and vegetables should be a high priority while foods containing fats should not even find their way to your priority list. Onions and other raw food has been proven to be advantageous to diabetes sufferers as these food has been proven to reduce blood sugar.

What to avoid that can worsen diabetes.

The following can lead to the development of diabetes or worsen diabetes:

- Eggs
- Tobacco
- Eating sugar
- Cheese
- Coffee
- Cow's milk
- Meat
- Greasy foods
- White flour products
- Rancid nut or seed
- Too much vegetable oil
- Gluten foods such as wheat, barley, and oats

Here's Dr. Sebi's natural food guide for more food you can rely on.

Natural herbs to help with diabetes:

The best way to ease your diabetes situation is to exercise a lot. This act helps with blood circulation to keep you away from a visit to the doctor.

- Black walnut, Echinacea, burdock root, and buchu help alleviate diabetes
- Huckleberry improves the production of insulin
- Dandelion root helps to reduce blood sugar
- Cedar berries gives the pancreas needed strength

Dr. Sebi natural food guide is helpful for treating diabetes

The safest and easily accessible food for diabetic people are fresh raw vegetables, freshly made salad of raw vegetables such as plum tomatoes, cabbage and lettuce seasoned with seeded yellow lemon juice. Totally avoid meat, bread, cooked vegetables and processed junk foods. Raw food should be your breakfast, lunch and dinner.

Natural alkaline seeded raw fruits are highly advised. These fruits includes coconut water, pears, peaches, sour sop, and lemon juice which oxidizes the excess blood sugar in the body. You should as a matter of fact stay away from GMO seedless fruits as they are too sweet.

Chapter [2]

BEST NATURAL FOODS FOR LIVER HEALTH AND ALKALINE DIETS FROM DR. SEBI'S NUTRITIONAL FOOD GUIDE LIST

The best foods for the healthy function of the liver is at the top of the best investments you can ever make for your body. The liver is a vital organ and it does more jobs than any other human organ. The liver handles a lot of chemically challenging activities with their own complexities. Basically, the liver is responsible for distributing numerous chemicals to intended places in order to provide energy. A diet that consists of clean foods is good for the health of the liver as this will keep it working optimally.

Here are some proven foods for liver and health nutrition.

Foods for good liver functionality:

The foods suggested for liver health are alkaline, natural, GMO-free and organic foods. They are rich in minerals and compliment the body's biological molecular structure.

Here are some potassium-rich foods for liver health:

- Banana
- Almond
- Kelp
- Dulse
- Prunes and
- Raisins

Water is inarguably the best food for liver health

- Divide your body weight by two and take that number in ounces of pure natural spring water.

Juices and raw fresh vegetables for liver health

- Dandelion greens
- Amaranth greens
- Rosemary
- Asparagus
- Okra
- Plum tomatoes
- Cabbage and

Fennel (see Dr. Sebi's nutritional guide for full list (https://www.amazon.com/dp/B07RXLZ8VN)).

Raw nuts is good for a healthy liver

- Brazil nuts
- Hazel nuts
- Walnuts and
- Almond

Fruit juices are excellent nutrients for liver function.

You can check out => (https://www.amazon.com/dp/B07RXLZ8VN) for full list of Dr. Sebi's approved fruit list

- Apple juice - fresh and natural
- Fresh prune juice
- Ginger juice
- Lemon juice

Why were the above foods chosen for liver health and functionality?

- Apples make the liver efficient in its processes
- Asparagus stimulates the liver function
- Dandelion helps to cleanse the liver
- Ginger contains eight compounds that defends the liver
- Lemon juice aids in carrying oxygen to the liver in a bid to get rid of all fatty buildup

- Prune juice flushes every impurity from the liver
- Rosemary helps rejuvenates a weak liver

Now that you know how important the liver is, here are more reasons why you should eat only foods that are best for its optimal function. The liver is a gland that is responsible for getting rid of toxins in the body. This is the reason why priority should be given to your liver's health and functionality as doing otherwise will deprive the liver of its ability to store and conserve energy. Because I am a staunch believer of the liver's health and optimal function, I will take this book beyond its original scope of healthy foods for the liver.

Herbs for good liver health and function:

- Bayberry
- Dandelion
- Lobelia
- Parsley and
- Yellow dock

Chapter [3]

EXCEPTIONAL STRATEGIES OF DR. SEBI'S HIGH BLOOD PRESSURE DIET, HOW TO LOWER SYMPTOMS OF HIGH BLOOD PRESSURE, AND WHAT CAUSES HYPERTENSION

What is high blood pressure?

If the walls of the arteries were to be clogged or packed with plagues, the flow of blood will become restricted as it pumps from the heart to the aorta, when the arteries creates pressure in a situation like this, the blood pressure becomes higher than it should be and this results into hypertension (high blood pressure).

Poor diet is the leading cause of high blood pressure in the United States as it has been reported that over 85 percent reported high blood pressure cases are rooted in poor diet. More than any other race in the United States, African Americans reported more cases of having a high blood pressure. High blood pressure is a channel to other diseases such as kidney diseases, strokes, scarlet fever, large heart, typhoid fever, artery coronary diseases and tonsillitis. These diseases are rampant among African Americans who have a hypertensive health history.

What is considered to be high blood pressure?

To be certain of your blood pressure, you will need a blood pressure gauge for accuracy. This gauge is often called a sphygmomanometer and it records two basic types of information: the first being systolic which is the higher reading while the second is diastolic which is the lower reading.

Consequently, the diastolic high blood pressure is less worrisome than the systolic high blood pressure readings as the systolic shows the pressure of the blood built as it is being pumped through the passage ways in the arteries to the aorta. The blood pressure is definitely high when your systolic reading is high as a result of the artery walls being clogged thereby limiting blood flows. A normal systolic high blood pressure reading is usually between 120 – 150 millimeters. On the other hand, a high reading is 140/190; the indication of a systolic high blood pressure reading is over 180/115.

What causes high blood pressure?

High blood pressure is caused when the blood flowing to the arteries is high due to the consumption of foods that are capable of clogging the wall of the arteries. An act which results in a pressure through the arteries during the distribution of blood flow. Blood is pumped by the heart to the aorta then the arteries. Peradventure the walls of the arteries become narrow and hardened due to excessive plague caused by poor eating habits, the flow of blood in the passageway of the arteries suppresses. Worthy of note is the fact that as an individual gets older, the arteries gets hardened bit by bit and a bad diet will triple the possibility of a high blood pressure.

Some of the numerous causes of high blood pressure:

Asides clogged arteries, high blood pressure can also be cause by poor blood circulation. Synthetic drugs, processed foods and unhealthy behavior patterns also cause high blood pressure.

These behavioral pattern includes the following:

- Bad diet
- Tobacco intake
- Stress
- Excess coffee intake
- Fried and processed foods
- Over-eating
- Aging

Symptoms of High Blood Pressure:

According to Dr. Sebi, high blood pressure symptoms can be likened to "navy seal snipers" as there are no signs that a person's blood pressure is high. The few noticeable pointers of high blood pressure has always been difficulty in breathing, blurry vision, rapid pulses and incessant headache.

My mother when alive had high blood pressure, she once told me that her blood pressure symptoms are dizziness and that her pulse gets fast often. But, because high blood pressure symptoms are not always perceptible, it was given a nick name "the navy seal sniper killer."

Dr. Sebi High blood pressure diet:

- Every high blood pressure drug in the market imitates water. This is why it is important for you as an individual to drink a lot of clean water. For this to be effective, you will need to divide your weight by 2 and drink that much water daily. Why that much water? You may ask. Well, water thins the blood and makes passing through the arteries easy.

- Taking five different types of fruits (vegetables included) a day will prevent the arteries from getting clogged as a result of excess plague deposits. Fruits and vegetables that contains a high percentage of antioxidant protects the artery walls from plague deposits. Such fruits include cabbage, tomatoes, oranges, seeded grapes and peaches.

- Foods that are rich in potassium helps to reduce recurrent high blood pressure as it expels excess sodium from the body. Red potatoes contain a good amount of potassium.

- Fiber containing fruits are also of high benefit to high blood pressure sufferers as itwill lower the blood pressure while removing wastes from the artery walls at the same time.

High blood pressure after eating:

Food related high blood pressure knowledge is important as having no knowledge of what foods to eat and the ones to avoid is detrimental to the blood pressure level. No one wants to get a high blood pressure from eating like everybody else. Here are some food to avoid:

- Avoid overeating even the healthiest of food.

- Avoid salty foods as much as possible as they transform into plaque in the artery walls. In essence, avoid sodas, baking soda, soy sauce and meat tenderizers.
- Never eat canned foods.
- Eliminate dairy products such as sodium, cheese and alcohol from your diet.
- Do not eat in the evening
- Avoid every other type of rice except wild and brown

Dr. Sebi High blood pressure medication (natural herbs):

These herbs are recommended by Dr. Sebi as they help to open the blood vessels, open the artery walls and eliminate plaques from the wall of the arteries. These herbs contain natural alkaline and are high in minerals. These are not hearsays, they have been medically proved to be effective as blood pressure medication. These herbals are usually high in iron, some of these herbs include;

- Fennel
- Oregano
- Basil
- Yellow dock

- Black cohosh
- Cayenne

Chapter [4]

Dr. Sebi Electric Food List

DR. SEBI FRUIT LIST

- Apples
- Bananas
- Berries
- Cantaloupe
- Cherries
- Currants
- Dates
- Figs
- Grapes
- Limes
- Mango
- Melons

- Orange
- Papayas
- Peaches
- Pears
- Plums
- Prickly Pear
- Prunes
- Rasins
- Soft Jelly Coconuts
- Soursoups
- Tamarind

DR. SEBI VEGETABLE LIST

- Amaranth
- Arame
- Avocado
- Bell Pepper
- Chayote
- Cherry and Plum Tomato
- Cucumber
- Dandelion Greens
- Dulse
- Garbanzo Beans
- Hijiki
- Izote flower and leaf
- Kale
- Lettuce except iceberg
- Mushrooms except Shitake

- Nopales
- Nori
- Okra
- Olives
- Onions
- Purslane Verdolaga
- Squash
- Tomatillo
- Turnip Greens
- Wakame
- Watercress
- Wild Arugula
- Zucchini

DR. SEBI HERB LIST

- Basil
- Cayenne
- Dill
- Onion powder
- Oregano
- Pure sea salt

ALKALINE SUGARS AND SWEETENERS

- Date Sugar from dried dates
- 100% Pure Agave Syrup from cactus

DR SEBI HERBAL TEAS

- Burdock
- Chamomile
- Elderberry
- Fennel
- Ginger
- Red Raspberry
- Tila

DR. SEBI ALKALINE GRAINS

- Amaranth
- Fonio
- Kamut
- Quinoa
- Rye
- Spelt
- Tef
- Wild Rice

DR SEBI FOOD LIST OF SPICES AND SEASONINGS

- Achiote
- Basil
- Bay Leaf
- Cayenne
- Cloves
- Dill
- Habanero
- Onion Powder
- Oregano
- Powdered Granulated Seaweed
- Pure Sea Salt
- Sage
- Savory

- Sweet Basil
- Tarragon
- Thyme
-

NOTE FROM THE AUHOR

High blood pressure is beatable by anyone who is dedicated to this newly discovered healthy lifestyle. People who have adhered to these simple things have a proven record of triumph. With the information in the article, you are on your way to beating high blood pressure. Always remember to check your blood level regularly, eat a healthy diet and exercise regularly.

Lastly, as one of my most favorable readers, your feedback is of the utmost importance to my book. I am always resolute to offer the best experience for my readers, and your input helps me to define that experience. That being said, if you could take a minute to post a REVIEW on this book here on Amazon, I would so much appreciate it.

Hope to see you again soon!

Contact the Author

It is always a great pleasure to know about your candid opinion on each book I put out.

For questions, suggestions and contribution, kindly reach out to me on carinchendry@gmail.com

Thank you for believing in me. I look forward to your messages.

Carin

CHECK OUT MY OTHER SIMILAR BOOKS:

DR. SEBI INSPIRED DETOX NUTRITIONAL GUIDE:
Adopting An Alkaline Diet Through Dr. Sebi Approved Food List And Herbs

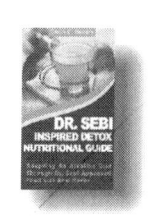

https://www.amazon.com/dp/B07RXLZ8VN

DR. SEBI APPROVED HERBS: *Cleanse, Heal and Revitalize Your Body With Dr. Sebi Herbs by Adopting an Alkaline Diet through Dr. Sebi*

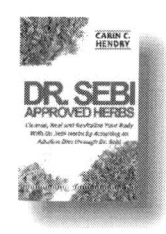

https://www.amazon.com/dp/B07TYPSRFF

DR. SEBI FASTING: *A royal road to Healing by fasting and losing weight through Dr. Sebi Alkaline Diet (Plant-Based Diet, mucus less diet)*

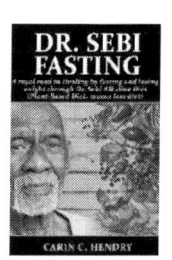

https://www.amazon.com/dp/B07ZC9XG6Y

DR. SEBI APPROVED 12 DAY SMOOTHIE DETOX GUIDE: *12 Delicious Dr. Sebi Smoothie Recipes to Cleanse and Revitalize Your Body by Following an Alkaline Diet Through Dr. Sebi Nutritional Guide*
https://www.amazon.com/dp/B07SQR1KK7

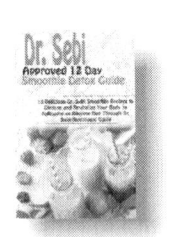

DR. SEBI DETOX CLEANSE: *Revitalize Yourself With Dr. Sebi Mucus Cleansing Alkaline Diet By Adopting An Alkaline Diet Through Dr. Sebi*

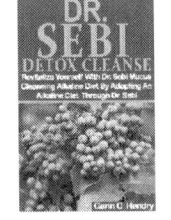

https://www.amazon.com/dp/B07XJCTLW1

DR. SEBI DIET - 2 in 1 MANUSCRIPT: *A Complete Guide On Dr. Sebi's Alkaline Recipes and Delicious Smoothies Using The Sebian Food List And Ingredients*

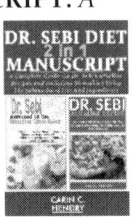

https://www.amazon.com/dp/B07XVWHGFM

DR. SEBI CURE FOR HERPES: *A Simple Guide On How To Cure Herpes Simplex Virus Using Dr. Sebi Alkaline Diet Eating Method*

https://www.amazon.com/dp/B07WVR8H6W

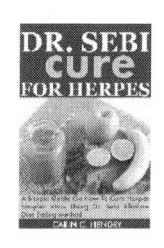

DIRTY LAZY KETO: *The Complete Beginner Guide On Ketogenic Diet For Weight Loss Using Keto Diet Recipes*

https://www.amazon.com/dp/B07SRKBLBM

KETOSIS STRIPS: *The Complete User Guide To Using Keto Test Strips To Measure Ketone Levels In Urine And Blood And Getting Into Ketosis Faster*

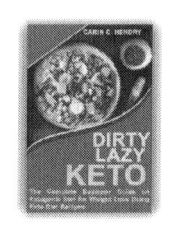

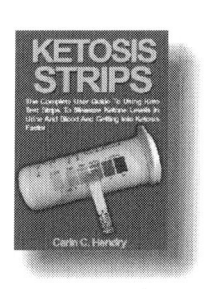

https://www.amazon.com/dp/B07S6GQFTL

Thanks For Reading

Made in the USA
Columbia, SC
05 November 2019